Vegan baby

A guide to complementary feeding

For vegans between the ages of 4 and 12 months

Christian Koeder, MSc

To Jade

Contents

Caveat emptor

For legal reasons, it must be stated that the recommendations in this book are not intended to replace medical advice or even medical treatment. Please be sure to discuss all these recommendations with your pediatrician. However, also be aware that your pediatrician is unlikely to be an expert in nutrition, or even vegan nutrition.

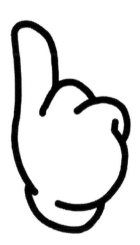

"It's not enough to know, you also have to apply."
Johann Wolfgang von Goethe

Preface

Vegan nutrition for babies is still a contentious issue for many, causing a lot of uncertainty, or even instilling fear. Can a completely vegan diet really be suitable for children and even babies? In other words, can a completely vegan diet provide all the necessary nutrients which are needed to allow the baby to grow normally and develop healthily, both physically and mentally? The answer is yes ... but certain nutrients should be paid attention to – most importantly vitamin B12. In other words, a vegan baby's diet should be "well-planned". What does "well-planned" mean? This booklet will explain.

But wouldn't it be safer to err on the side of caution and give your baby a "normal", i.e. a non-vegetarian diet? The answer is: No, not really ... as long as the vegan diet is well-planned. Nothing suggests that a well-planned vegan diet is any less safe than a typical "Western" (i.e. a not very well-planned) diet – or even than a very well-planned non-vegan diet. There is also no evidence that a typical "Western" or other non-vegan diet would have a more beneficial effect on a baby's long-term health and life expectancy compared to a well-planned vegan diet.

All recommendations in this book are evidence-based. That means that they are based on what is known from scientific studies, including the most recent scientific studies. These recommendations are also supported by years of personal experience.

Some basic questions and answers

Question: Can serious nutritional deficiencies occur in both vegan and non-vegan babies?

Answer: Yes.

Question: Is the risk of serious nutritional deficiencies with a poorly-planned vegan diet higher for the baby than with a typical "Western", non-vegan diet?

Answer: Yes, quite likely so. Especially in terms of vitamin B12 deficiency.

Question: Wouldn't it be safer to compromise and to raise your baby on an ovo-lacto-vegetarian rather than a vegan diet?

Answer: That depends. An unplanned ovo-lacto-vegetarian diet is quite probably safer for babies than an unplanned vegan diet. However, a well-planned vegan diet is probably safer than an unplanned ovo-lacto-vegetarian diet and at least as safe as a well-planned ovo-lacto-vegetarian diet.

Question: Should non-vegan complementary feeding also be well-planned?

Answer: Yes. But that is not the topic of this book.

Question: What are the health benefits of well-planned vegan complementary feeding compared to a typical non-vegan, "Western" diet for babies?

Answer: That is not entirely clear. It is, however, likely that a healthy, i.e. a well-planned vegan (or other plant-based) diet before and during pregnancy, during breastfeeding as well once the baby starts eating "real" food can have a positive impact on the child's lifelong health and life expectancy.

As mentioned above, how well-planned vegan complementary feeding can be accomplished is shown in this book.

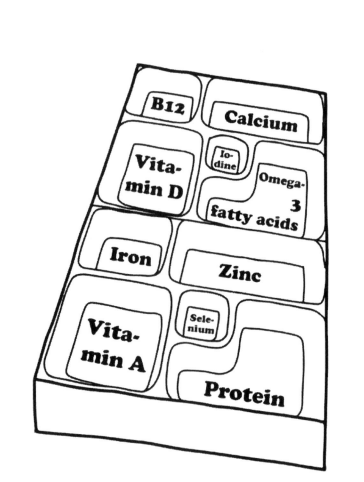

The ten key nutrients in a vegan diet

1) **Vitamin B12**[1–9]

2) **Calcium**[2,3,5,9–11]

3) **Vitamin D**[4,9,12–15]

4) **Iodine**[4,5,9,16–18]

5) **Omega-3 fatty acids**[2,3,9]

6) **Iron**[1–4,9,19–22]

7) **Zinc**[1–3,9,19–21,23–25]

8) **Selenium**[26–30]

9) **Vitamin A**[2]

10) **Protein**[1,2,9,12,19,22,31]

What you should know:
The ten nutrients listed above are of interest to vegans of all ages. When planning your baby's diet, however, paying attention to these is particularly important.[32] Unsurprisingly, paying attention to these nutrients is also especially important for pregnant and breastfeeding women.[33–36]

Official non-vegetarian recommendations for complementary feeding in Germany

The three purees ("infant cereal") for babies: a German tradition

In Germany there is – at least officially – a practically universal recommendation for complementary feeding, which is called the "three purees". The three types of puree and their exact composition are not just based on nutrient content but also, simply, on tradition in Germany. So, if you would like to follow the "three purees" concept, it is not important to stick to the exact food composition of these purees as recommended, but instead to incorporate the equivalent vegan food groups. This way you can create vegan alternatives to the original versions.

Non-vegan foods in the traditional German recommendations[32] can simply be replaced by their vegan "counterparts" – and these vegan alternatives must provide the same essential nutrients.

The three traditional purees:

- **Puree One** (age: 4 to 6 months): vegetable, potato & meat puree (occasionally add some wheat noodles; at times use fatty fish instead of meat)
- **Puree Two** (age: 5 to 7 months): cereal & cow's milk puree
  (Cow's milk is generally recommended to be used only as an ingredient for baby cereal and not as a drink for babies.[2,32,37,38])
- **Puree Three** (age: 6 to 8 months): cereal & fruit puree

Additional suggestions – also suitable for vegan babies

Tip: Don't add salt*,[2,12,32,39] artificial flavors, sugar or syrup[2,12,32,39] to complementary foods.

(* The technical term for normal table salt is sodium chloride. The sodium in sodium chloride can increase blood pressure, which in the long-term can damage the arteries. Sodium is also found in baking powder or baking soda, for example. Therefore, it is best not to use baking powder or baking soda for complementary food either.)

Tip: Contrary to earlier assumptions, it is not necessary to avoid certain foods – such as nuts or wheat – in complementary feeding in order to reduce the risk of your baby developing allergies.[2,12,32,39–41]

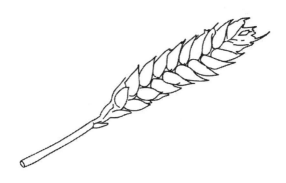

Vegan complementary feeding: take vegan ingredients.

First option: the three vegan purees

As mentioned earlier, it is not the three purees in and of themselves that are important, but the nutrient-rich food groups used to make them. Let's look at the vegan versions of the three purees mentioned in the last chapter.

- **Puree One** (age: 4 to 6 months): vegetable, potato & legume puree (occasionally add some wheat noodles; add vitamin B12 to your baby's diet – *see page 14*)
- **Puree Two** (age: 5 to 7 months): cereal & soy milk puree
  (Soy milk is recommended to be used only as an ingredient for baby cereal and not as a drink for babies; the soy milk should be fortified with calcium and it should not contain any salt. Preferably it should contain as little added sugar as possible.)
- **Puree Three** (age: 6 to 8 months): cereal & fruit puree

Second option: just pay attention to the food groups.

The food groups for vegan babies

Except for breast milk, the vegan food groups for babies are just like the vegan food groups for adults. The vegan food groups for babies are:

Breast milk,[36] fruit, vegetables, legumes,[39,42] and grains[43,44] as well as nuts or seeds, and oils – plus supplements.[45]

The vegan food groups for babies

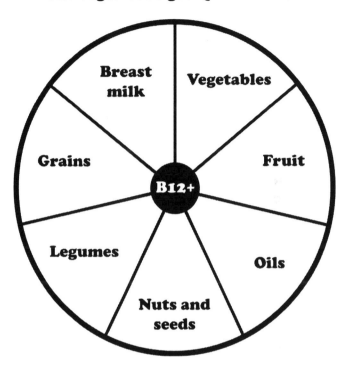

Vegan complementary feeding: the food groups

B12+: Vitamin B12 supplement, plus further supplements if required (*see page 14*)

Figure adapted from "Supplemental Figure 2. The VegPlate for infants (6 to 12 months)" by Baroni et al (2019)[46]

Tip: Mix it up. Alternate different types of fruit, vegetables, grains, legumes, and nuts or seeds.[2,32,42,47]

Tip: Healthy, unrefined plant foods contain large amounts of fiber and generally have a lower caloric density (i.e. less calories per volume) than animal-source foods. However, a baby's or a toddler's stomach is small. Therefore, care should be taken to ensure that vegan complementary foods are not too high in fiber and that a sufficient amount of high-calorie foods are fed to your baby (*see page 23*).[5,45]

Suitable oils[12]
Which oils are best? For example, extra virgin (cold-pressed) olive oil, cold-pressed canola (rapeseed) oil, or cold-pressed flaxseed (linseed) oil. Use olive oil for cooking, i.e. if you heat the oil at all.

Daily recommendation:
- approximately 2 teaspoons of canola oil
or
- approximately ½ teaspoon of flaxseed oil
  + 1½ teaspoons of olive oil

Do not use too much oil for your baby's food because oil is made up of 100% fat, and it contains no protein. If too much oil is eaten, this could displace high-protein foods in your baby's diet.[46]

What should your baby drink?

Suitable drinks[12,32]

- Tap water or still (non-carbonated), bottled mineral water*
- Carrot juice (small amounts; without honey[2,48–50])
- Unsweetened herbal tea or fruit tea (small amounts;[51] no fennel tea[2])

* In some countries the label on mineral water will state if it is suitable for babies. If this is not the case, look for the sodium (Na) content (should be less than 200 mg/liter) and the sulphate (SO_4) content (should be less than 250 mg/liter).

No coffee, black tea, green tea, white tea, mate tea, energy drinks, or cola or other carbonated soft drinks should be given to infants.[51]

Tips regarding tap water

- Let the tap water run until the water comes out cold. This way you will avoid the water stored in the pipes overnight for example.
- In some countries it is recommended to boil tap or bottled water (and let it cool down again!) before giving it to babies. Boiling water will kill the bacteria in the water.
- Do not use tap water for your baby if your building has lead pipes (water pipes made out of lead).
- Use water from domestic wells only after having it tested and having been assured that it is suitable for babies.

How often should your baby drink water?

Babies do not need to drink water at all until about two months after they have started eating complementary foods. That is, babies need to drink water at the earliest from the age of six months. The World Health Organization (WHO) actually recommends that babies should not drink water before they are six months old.[52]

There are exceptions: In case of fever or diarrhea, your baby's need for fluids is increased, and your baby should drink some water.

How should your baby drink?

- Preferably from a mug or a cup[32]
- It is best to avoid giving your baby a bedtime bottle,[53–57] or allowing them to always have a bottle with them to suckle on.

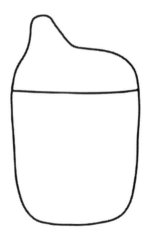

Which supplements are recommended for babies in general?

The recommendations in this section are not specific to vegan babies. Your family doctor or pediatrician will inform you about the recommendations in your country. In Germany there is a practically universal recommendation regarding supplements for babies (*see below*).

In **Germany*** practically all babies receive the following three supplements:

- **Vitamin K** … which is important in blood clotting to prevent excessive bleeding.[2,58]
- **Vitamin D** … which is important for healthy bones, a strong immune system, and good general health.[2,12,59,60]
- **Fluoride** … which is recommended only once teeth begin to appear. Fluoride protects against caries by hardening the uppermost layer of the teeth (the enamel).[59,61]

* In the **United States**,[62,63] the **United Kingdom**,[64] and **Canada**[65–67] (for example, but also in many other countries[68,69]) these recommendations are very similar (*see next page*).

Regarding the correct amounts, please follow the advice of your family doctor or pediatrician. The following **dosages** are generally recommended.

Vitamin K	
Germany	3 x 2 mg; on the day of birth, at 4–6 days old, and at 1 month old; as drops[70,71]
USA/ Canada	1 x 0.5–1.0 mg; on the day of birth; intramuscular injection[62,63,67,70]
UK	Vitamin K drops or injections are recommended; on the day of birth; variable local policies[72]
A health care professional will administer this supplement.	

Vitamin D	
Germany	400–500 IU* per day; from the age of 1 week; as dissolving tablets or drops[9,71,73–77]
USA/ Canada	400 IU per day; from the first few days of life[62,65,78–80]
UK	340–400 IU per day; from birth[64,81–83]
* IU = international units; vitamin D conversion: 400 IU = 10 µg; µg = microgram = one millionth of a gram	

Can your baby get enough vitamin D from sunshine?

If you live in a country with plenty of sunshine, relatively close to the equator – let's say in Ecuador, Mexico, or Thailand, for example – your baby (and you) can make enough vitamin D from sunshine if the skin is regularly exposed to the sun year-round, and your baby and you might not need vitamin D supplements.[84,85] But this is in conflict with the widely-given recommendation that babies should not be exposed to direct sunlight because doing so

10

could increase the risk for faster skin ageing and skin cancer much later in life.[68,86] Based on current evidence, it seems that a small amount of careful sun exposure can be beneficial and that babies should not avoid sunshine completely.[87–89] However, sunburn must be avoided at all costs.[90] Sunshine can be an alternative to vitamin D supplements if such supplements are not available to you. But even if you and your baby live in a sunny part of the world, a vitamin D supplement with 400 IU per day would probably be best.[91]

Fluoride	
Germany	Usually 0.25 mg per day; from the age of 6 months; as a tablet*[71]
USA	A supplement (0.25 mg per day) if water is not fluoridated; from 6 months[62,92]
Canada	Flouride supplements are not generally recommended.[66,93]
UK	A small smear of fluoride toothpaste twice daily[64,82]

* Fluoride tablets should only be given if the local tap water contains less than 0.3 mg/L** fluoride.[63,94–97] Your family doctor/pediatrician prescribing the fluoride tablets should know if this is the case.

In Germany fluoride levels in water are generally low. In other countries or regions the water supply is often fluoridated.[66,98]

** mg/liter of water = parts per million (ppm)

Fluoride from toothpaste, supplements, or tap water?
Often fluoride toothpaste is recommended for babies instead of fluoride supplements.[57,64,99] Care should be taken so that the baby will not swallow the toothpaste, and only a very small amount ("a smear") of toothpaste should be used.[57,100]

What about iron?
Sometimes **iron supplements** or **iron-fortified foods**[2,101] are recommended from the age of around four months until enough iron-rich foods are eaten.[80,102] However, using iron supplements in the absence of iron deficiency anemia is controversial,[2,81,82,102–108] because iron is a prooxidant and excess iron can promote inflammation and infections.[109,110] So, it is best to discuss with your family doctor or pediatrician[101] and to use iron supplements only if necessary. Legumes are a rich source of iron, especially if consumed together with a good source of vitamin C. It is widely recommended that the first complementary foods given should be rich in iron.[2] Therefore, legumes (which are iron-rich) should be one of the first complementary foods given. In this way legumes can replace red meat as an iron source.[111–113]

What about other supplements?
In addition, in the United Kingdom, babies often receive **vitamin A** and **vitamin C** supplements from the age of six months.[64,81,83] This however does not seem necessary[81] if your baby consumes good sources of vitamin C and beta-carotene (provitamin A[51]) – ideally daily or nearly every day.

What if your baby is fed infant formula?

If breast feeding is not possible and your baby is getting infant formula instead of breast milk, vitamin D supplements are likely not necessary (depending on how much formula in consumed),[85,91] because infant formula is already fortified with vitamin D and many other nutrients. To avoid excessive intake of any nutrients, please discuss any combination of formula feeding and supplements with your family doctor or pediatrician.

Tip: Be sure to attend all of the regular medical check-ups (early detection examinations) at your pediatrician's practice with your baby.[3,114] There are many (fortunately very rare) diseases that have to be detected early on in order to be treated appropriately. Your pediatrician will also supervise the "normal", i.e. healthy growth and development of your baby.[115,116] Well-nourished vegan babies do not grow and develop differently (faster, more slowly, or differently in any other way) compared to other children.[2,5,9,10,117–123] Your family doctor or pediatrician (i.e. a medical doctor), and not anyone else (nutritionist, alternative practitioner, nurse, helpful people on internet forums, etc.) is the right person to monitor the healthy development of your baby and to make therapy suggestions in case of health problems.

Important: A vegan diet for babies and children must be well-planned – as described in this little book. A well-planned vegan diet (as compared to a typical "Western" diet for children) can probably have beneficial effects on your child's health throughout his or her life and can probably reduce the risk of illness later in life.[39,115,124,125]

Which supplements are recommended for vegan babies?

First, the same supplements that are recommended for non-vegan babies (general recommendations – *see previous chapter*) are also suitable for vegan babies, i.e. vitamin K, vitamin D, and – as soon as teeth appear and depending on where you live – fluoride.[20]

Note: The vitamin D3 in most common vitamin D supplements is not vegan. It is produced from lanolin, which is extracted from sheep's wool. However, the amounts of sheep's wool used for this purpose are extremely small.

Second, vegan babies, starting at the age of four to six months, should receive a **vitamin B12 supplement**:[64,83]

- about 5 (to 10) μg of vitamin B12 per day[2,9,20,45,76,82,107,126–129]

If you live in Europe, an example of a vegan supplement could be 1/8 to 1/4 of a tablet of the supplement "Vegan Society VEG 1". This chewable tablet can be cut into pieces with a knife and the pieces can be crushed into a "powder" or small crumbs. These small tablet pieces can then be mixed into the complementary food. The "Vegan Society VEG 1" supplement also contains iodine (*see next page*), and several other nutrients.

Third, vegan babies should receive an additional **iodine supplement**,[9,16,126] if (<u>and only if</u>) your baby at this stage does not drink a lot of breast milk anymore.

Whether or not an iodine supplement should be given and what exact amount of iodine would be ideal depends on how much breast milk the baby still drinks every day:

- If your baby **does not drink any breast milk** at all anymore: Either use soy-based infant formula (which is fortified with nutrients, including iodine), <u>or</u> use a supplement with approx. 80 µg of iodine per day[16,33,130–133] (60 to 130 µg per day, not more).[76,130]
- If your baby drinks **less than 500 ml** (~17 US fluid ounces) of breast milk per day: Use a supplement with approx. 30 µg of iodine per day.[16,33,130,131,134,135] (If you live in Europe this could be approx. 1/8 to 1/4 of a tablet of "Vegan Society VEG 1".)
- If your baby still drinks **around 500 ml** (~17 US fluid ounces) of breast milk per day: No additional iodine is needed.[45,46,134,135] Optionally, you may use a supplement of approx. 20 to 30 µg of iodine per day.[130] (Again, if you live in Europe this could be approx. 1/8 to 1/4 of a tablet of "Vegan Society VEG 1".)
- If your baby still drinks **around 1000 ml** (~34 US fluid ounces) of breast milk per day: It is best not to add any additional iodine to your baby's diet, i.e. <u>no iodine supplement should be given</u>.[16,33,45,46,134,135]

Tip: Sometimes nori – the seaweed used to make sushi – is recommended as a source of iodine for babies. If you use nori as a complementary food for your baby,[1,126,136,137] you should not give your baby more than half a sheet (~1 gram; ~0.04 ounces) of nori per day, and you should <u>not</u> give your baby nori every day. On days when your baby has eaten nori, he or she should not receive an iodine supplement or iodine-containing supplement (such as "Vegan Society VEG 1").

Supplements for vegan babies		
Nutrient	**Amount**	**Age**
Vitamin B12	5 µg daily	Starting at 4 to 6 months
Iodine	Depending on the amount of breast milk consumed (*see previous page*)	
Vitamin K	According to your family doctor's or pediatrician's recommendation (*see page 9*)	
Vitamin D*		
Fluoride		
* Your baby should not receive more than 25–30 µg (1000–1200 IU) of vitamin D daily, unless otherwise prescribed by your doctor.[68,73,138,139]		

Caution: Parents should understand that a severe vitamin B12 deficiency can be extremely dangerous for their baby.[2,140–143] This could – in the worst case – even result in death. So, please do follow the advice above, and make sure your baby gets all the vitamin B12 they need.

Caution: Not only too little iodine, but also too much iodine must be avoided at all costs.

Tip: All supplements are best discussed with your pediatrician,[5] although most medical doctors do not have extensive knowledge of vegan nutrition.[144] However, they will know what your country's guidelines regarding vitamin D supplementation for babies are. Maybe you will find it useful to show them this booklet.

Tip: Most nutritional scientists – including renowned nutrition experts – do not possess detailed and specialized knowledge of how to plan vegan diets, especially for babies. This also applies to most nutritionists in general (many nutritionists do not have university degrees in nutrition science). Especially when it comes to feeding babies, it is very important not to rely on (i.e. not to fall for) misinformation. Therefore, information regarding vegan baby nutrition is best obtained from nutritional scientists who specialize in the field of vegan nutrition.

Supplements: Use supplements in the form of chewable tablets (nicely ground up/crushed) or drops that you can add to food. Or you can put drops directly into your baby's mouth,[51] or you can let your baby suckle the drops from your fingertip, or you can put drops on a teaspoon.[82]

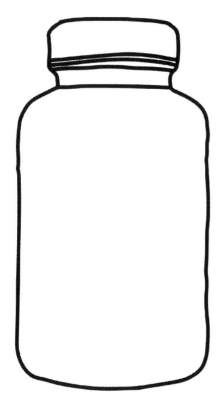

Important: Keep all supplements out of reach of babies and children.

Supplements for breastfeeding women

It is highly recommended that breastfeeding vegan women optimize their nutrient intake. This also means paying attention to the ten key nutrients in vegan diets, and taking the appropriate supplements – as needed (*see below*).[2,33,34,126,134,145–148]

- **Vitamin B12:** Take a supplement with 2–5 μg (more is OK) twice per day, or 10–200 μg once a day.[45,128,129,149]
- **Calcium:** Consume calcium-rich foods, for example calcium-fortified soy milk/soy yogurt, bok choy, kale, broccoli, Collard greens, tofu made with calcium, or calcium-rich water.
- **Vitamin D:** Use a supplement with 15–25 μg (600–1000 IU) per day.[45,149–151]
- **Iodine:** Use a supplement with 150–250 μg per day,[33,76,130,149,152] and use iodized salt for cooking (but not for your baby's food[2,12]).
- **Omega-3 fatty acids:** Eat omega-3 fatty acid-rich foods, for example, 2 tablespoons of canola oil, or 2 teaspoons of flaxseed oil, or 2 tablespoons of chia seeds per day,[125] and take a vegan supplement with approx. 200 mg of DHA* per day (or every other day) – in the form of microalgae oil or microalgae oil supplements.[2,12,45,153,154]
  (* DHA is a long-chain omega-3 fatty acid, and is short for docosahexaenoic acid. Note that an excessive intake of omega-3 fatty acids can lead to small, point-shaped bruises in the skin called petechiae. Should this occur, reduce the amount of omega-3-rich foods you consume.)

- **Iron, zinc, and protein:** Eat grains, legumes, and some nuts & seeds daily.
- **Selenium:** If you live in an area with selenium-rich soils (including, generally speaking, the United States, Canada, Venezuela, and some areas of China[155,156]), you do not need a selenium supplement. If you live in an area with low-selenium soils (most of the world), consider taking a supplement with 50–60 µg of selenium (selenomethionine) per day[76,157–159] – or eat one Brazil nut per day.[160,161] Soils in Europe are generally low in selenium, and soils in New Zealand are generally very low in selenium.[156]
- **Vitamin A:** Consume beta-carotene-rich foods, for example carrots, carrot juice, pumpkin, orange-fleshed sweet potatoes, red peppers, green leafy vegetables, papayas, mangos, or apricots.

If you live in Europe, you could cover your vitamin B12, vitamin D, iodine, and selenium needs by taking 1 to 1½ tablets of the supplement "Vegan Society VEG 1" per day. If you take it in two doses per day, this will optimize the amount of vitamin B12 absorbed.

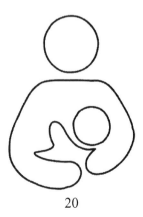

Good sources of the ten key nutrients

A basic **question** that many people, including many nutritionists, will ask – you or themselves – when it comes to raising your child on a vegan diet is:

How can a vegan diet provide the same essential nutrients which in traditional complementary feeding are supplied by animal-source foods, i.e. meat, fish, dairy, and eggs?

The **answer** is: With vegan complementary feeding attention should be paid to supply adequate amounts of the ten key nutrients discussed earlier. In the following table you can see the ten key nutrients and their respective vegan sources.

Nutrient	Supplied by ...
Vitamin B12	... breast milk[146,162] (the breastfeeding woman must consume enough vitamin B12 – *see page 19*), and starting at the age of 4 to 6 months, additionally a vitamin B12 supplement.[45,116]
Calcium	... breast milk, and starting at the age of 4 to 6 months, additionally calcium-fortified soy milk (as an ingredient in complementary foods).[3,163]
Vitamin D	... a supplement – and depending on where you live and the time of the year – additionally sunshine (as well as breast milk and possibly vegan fortified foods).

Nutrient	Supplied by ...
Iodine	... breast milk[16,33,134,135] (the breastfeeding woman must consume enough iodine – *see page 19*), and as soon as the amount of breast milk consumed is quite small, a supplement.
Omega-3 fatty acids	... breast milk, and starting at the age of 4 to 6 months, additionally small amounts of cold-pressed canola or flaxseed oil (DHA via breast milk[2]).
Iron	... breast milk, and starting at the age of 4 to 6 months, especially legumes[39,116,164] (often iron-fortified cereal is also recommended[2,22,32,39,165,166]).
Zinc	... breast milk, and starting at the age of 4 to 6 months, additionally legumes, and some nut or seed butters.[45,116]
Selenium*	... breast milk,[29,159,167–175] and starting at the age of 4 to 6 months, additionally legumes, and nut or seed butters; possibly a small additional amount from a supplement: 5 µg per day (up to 15 µg per day, not more!)[29,157] * In areas with selenium-rich soils (including the United States,[176] Canada, Venezuela, and some areas of China[155,167,173,174]) no selenium-containing supplements should be given.

Nutrient	Supplied by ...
Vitamin A	... breast milk, and starting at the age of 4 to 6 months, additionally orange and green vegetables, red bell peppers, mangos, papayas, or apricots (for example) – these are rich in beta-carotene (provitamin A).
Protein	... breast milk, and starting at the age of 4 to 6 months, additionally legumes, grains, and nut or seed butters.[12]
All other essential nutrients are easily obtained from the typical vegan food groups (*see page 5*).	

And how does your baby get enough calories?[12,19]

Our bodies obtain calories from the following nutrients:

- Carbohydrates (mainly sugar and starch)
- Fats
- Protein
- (... and also, alcohol – but not for babies!)

The main sources of calories are carbohydrates and fats.

Vegan babies receive sufficient calories from the following foods:

- Breast milk
- Legumes + oil
- Nut or seed butters
- Grains
- Fruit
- Soy milk (as an ingredient in complementary foods)

Tip: For the most part refined grains (white pasta/rice/bread)[177] should be given instead of whole grains.[46] The reason is that whole grains contain a great deal of fiber and can therefore fill up the baby's small stomach too quickly. Peeled legumes[45,46] – soy foods[41] like tofu,[2,5,19] soy yogurt, soy milk,[2,178,179] soy flour, as well as red lentils, yellow peas, etc. – should also be used. Fruit and vegetables that are very rich in fiber should be pressed through a sieve to remove coarse fibers.[45,46]

Tip: Rice and rice products, including white rice and (even more so) brown rice, as well as rice milk, rice cakes, rice pasta, brown rice syrup, rice cereal, and rice-based infant foods can be relatively high in arsenic.[177,180–185] This seems to be less of an issue with rice-based infant formula.[184–187] This does not mean that you must avoid rice completely. But your baby's diet should be varied and an excessive intake of rice products should be avoided.[188]

Good sources of vitamin C

Vegan diets are typically high in vitamin C because many (but not all) fruits and vegetables are rich in this vitamin. Vitamin C increases the amount of iron that can be absorbed from plant foods. Iron is very important for babies. So, adding good sources of vitamin C to complementary foods is a good idea.

Good sources of vitamin C		
• Papaya	• Gooseberries	• Passion fruit
• Strawberries	• Raspberries	• Mamey sapote
• Lemon juice	• Blueberries	• Cashew apple
• Oranges	• Tangerines	• Durian
• Orange juice	• Cantaloupe	• Red peppers
• Kiwi	• Red currants	• Brussels sprouts
• Grapefruit	• Guava	• Kale
• Lychees	• Rambutan	• Broccoli
… and many other fruits and vegetables		

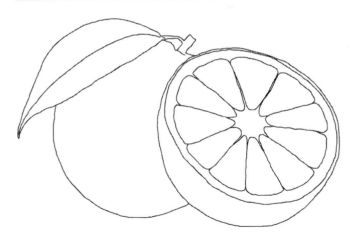

When should your baby start eating complementary foods?

Short answer: At the age of four, five, or six months.

Long answer:

- Your baby should consume only breast milk until at least four months of age.[2,12,32,189] Complementary feeding should therefore start at the earliest when your baby is four months old – and at the latest at six months old.[2,12,32,37,39,124,190] Breastfeeding should be continued at the same time.[12]

- If exclusive breastfeeding up to the age of four months is not possible, your baby should receive soy infant formula[2,3,126,191–198] – under no circumstances should breast milk be replaced by home-made formula or regular plant milks, such as soy milk, rice milk, oat milk, almond milk, coconut milk, or similar products.[199] If you consider the use of donor human milk, please seek the advice of a healthcare provider first, who can inform you about the potential risks and benefits.[200] Donor human milk should be pasteurized and should come from a human milk bank.[201]

- The exact point in time when an individual baby is ready for complementary foods varies and depends on a baby's individual development (for example, when he or she can eat from a spoon and when they show interest in new foods).[12,124]

- Ideally, your baby will continue to be breastfed up to the age of two years (or longer) – in addition to their regular diet.[39,202,203]

- Breastfeeding has many health benefits – not just for your baby but also for the breastfeeding mother.[204–207]

Important: Plant-based milks such as soy milk, rice milk, oat milk, almond milk, etc. have a different nutrient composition than cow's milk.[3,96,126,208] Soy milk is a good source of protein, but unlike cow's milk it does not provide vitamin B12 – unless the soy milk is fortified with this vitamin. Rice milk,[2,199,208–210] almond milk, and oat milk are low in protein and are not well-suited to a baby's nutrient needs.

Tip: It is best to eat together with your baby.[12]

Tip: It is best not to use food to comfort or reward your baby.[2,32,211,212]

Tip: Feed your baby slowly and patiently. Encourage your baby to eat, but do not force them. Talk to your baby and maintain eye contact.[203]

Tip: It is quite normal for a baby to vehemently reject some foods when trying them for the first time. This does not mean that your baby does not like this particular food.[124] A baby just needs time to become accustomed to tastes and textures of the plethora of other foods besides breast milk. You can simply offer this type of food again on another day.

Tip: At the age of six to eight months, feed your baby two to three meals per day, and at the age of nine to 12 months, three to four meals per day.[203]

Recipe ideas

In the following a few ideas for complementary food meals are presented. These are not real recipes – and you do not need real recipes. The aim here is to feed your baby foods from the different vegan food groups (*see page 5*) – either one food on its own, or several, pureed, mashed, shaped into little balls, …

- **Lentil balls:** Boil some sushi rice and some red (or yellow) lentils. Both should be nice and soft. Leave to cool, and by hand shape them into small balls. Instead of sushi rice you can also use potatoes or sweet potatoes.
- **Spelt & soy milk pancakes:** Mix equal amounts of whole grain spelt flour (or other flour) and soy milk (with calcium, without salt). Fry gently in some olive oil until golden brown. You can also replace a small amount of spelt flour with a little bit of soy flour. You can also blend a ripe banana into the pancake batter. (Basic recipe: ~half flour, half soy milk).
- **Vegetable waffles:** Finely grate some zucchini (courgettes) and carrot. Make a waffle dough from some flour, soy milk (with calcium, without salt), olive oil, and the grated vegetables. Bake in a waffle iron.
- **Avocado and bread:** Soft white or sourdough bread (without the crust or seeds) with some well-mashed avocado.

- **Finger food:**[12,32] Cooked potato, pasta (soft-boiled), vegetables (cooked; for example, carrot, pumpkin, broccoli, cauliflower), fruit (peeled: apple, pear, banana, peach, nectarine; berries; "filleted": orange, tangerine), avocado,[2,19] tofu (well-rinsed).[2]
- **Porridge:** For example, soy milk and oatmeal porridge, banana and millet porridge, semolina and apple porridge, ...
- **Baby hummus:**[19] Blend cooked chickpeas with a little tahini, fresh lemon juice and olive oil until very creamy (no salt).

Other suitable foods (examples):
Almond butter,[2] very soft white rice*, soy yogurt (fortified with calcium, no added sugar), iron-fortified vegan baby foods,[2,22,32,39] yellow (peeled) or green peas*, mung dal (peeled mung beans)*, tomato sauce*, cashew nut butter, peanut butter (100% peanuts, no salt), quinoa (very soft)*,[115] millet (very soft)*, buckwheat*, couscous*, ground flaxseeds[213] or chia seeds (pureed with other foods; no more than 1 teaspoon per day), nutritional yeast flakes,[45] pineapple, tahini (sesame seed butter), ground-up nuts (pureed with other foods), polenta*, red bell peppers*, mango, papaya, apricot, kiwi, cantaloupe, watermelon (without seeds), soft dried fruit (for example, figs, dates, unsulphured apricots), parsnips*, small quantities of kale*, pak choi* and other green leafy vegetables*,[2] small quantities of spices and herbs (for example, paprika, thyme, basil, cumin, ...)*.

* cooked

Functions of the ten key nutrients

The following table gives a quick overview of the most important functions of the above-mentioned key nutrients.

Nutrient	Function
Vitamin B12	Protection of nerve cells, the brain, the heart, and the arteries
Calcium	Building and maintenance of bones and teeth
Vitamin D	Absorption of calcium in the intestine, protection of bones, teeth, arteries, the brain, and the immune system
Iodine	Protection of the thyroid and the brain
Omega-3 fatty acids	Protection of the arteries, heart, brain, eyes, and all other organs
Iron	Oxygen transport in the blood and energy production (strength and vitality), physical growth and brain development, protection of the brain and the immune system
Zinc	Protection of the immune system, eyes, and skin, wound healing, sexual development and testosterone production, smell and taste perception
Selenium	Protection of the thyroid, the heart, and the immune system

Nutrient	Function
Vitamin A	Physical growth and brain development, protection of nerve cells, the skin and mucous membranes, the immune system, lungs, eyes, bones, and teeth
Protein	Building and maintenance of muscles and bones, protection of the immune system

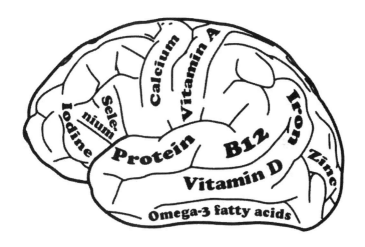

Thank you

Many thanks to the reader and to all who conscientiously help to inform the public about vegan nutrition and veganism. Many thanks to Benny, Bella, and Henri, Pete, Anne-Celine, Erik, Stephanie, Tony, Vroni, and all the others. Many thanks also to Ashley Hooper, Jon Active, Howard Strauss, Shari Leskowitz, Heather Russell (Vegan Society), Maria Andersson, Michael Zimmermann, ...

Author

Christian Koeder (*1979) has been a vegan since 1997. He holds degrees in nutritional sciences from the Justus Liebig University in Gießen, Germany (Bachelor of Science, Master of Science), and currently works as a researcher at the University of Applied Sciences in Münster, Germany, where he explores the connections between healthy plant-based eating, lifestyle change and health, and where he also teaches a college course on vegan nutrition.

The author is not a member of the Vegan Society, or any other organization, does not sell any supplements and has no financial, personal, or ideological ties to any manufacturers or vendors of supplements.

More info

Further information, for example, articles such as "How should vegan children grow?", can be found on: **christiankoeder.com**

References

1. Cofnas, N. Is vegetarianism healthy for children? *Critical reviews in food science and nutrition* **59,** 2052–2060; 10.1080/10408398.2018.1437024 (2019).
2. Fewtrell, M. *et al.* Complementary feeding: a position paper by the European Society for Paediatric Gastroenterology, Hepatology, and Nutrition (ESPGHAN) Committee on Nutrition. *Journal of pediatric gastroenterology and nutrition* **64,** 119–132; 10.1097/MPG.0000000000001454 (2017).
3. Scaglioni, S., Cosmi, V. de, Mazzocchi, A., Bettocchi, S. & Agostoni, C. in *Vegetarian and Plant-Based Diets in Health and Disease Prevention* (Elsevier2017), pp. 513–527.
4. Lubetzky, R., Mandel, D. & Mimouni, F. B. Vitamin and mineral supplementation of term infants: are they necessary? *World review of nutrition and dietetics* **108,** 79–85; 10.1159/000351489 (2013).
5. Ferrara, P. *et al.* Caring for Infants and Children Following Alternative Dietary Patterns. *The Journal of pediatrics* **187,** 339-340.e1; 10.1016/j.jpeds.2017.04.053 (2017).
6. Boran, P. *et al.* The impact of vitamin B12 deficiency on infant gut microbiota. *European journal of pediatrics*; 10.1007/s00431-019-03517-2 (2019).
7. Aguirre, J. A. *et al.* Compromiso neurológico grave por déficit de vitamina B12 en lactantes hijos de madres veganas y vegetarianas. *Archivos argentinos de pediatria* **117,** e420-e424; 10.5546/aap.2019.e420 (2019).
8. Irevall, T., Axelsson, I. & Naumburg, E. B12 deficiency is common in infants and is accompanied by serious neurological symptoms. *Acta paediatrica (Oslo, Norway : 1992)* **106,** 101–104; 10.1111/apa.13625 (2017).
9. Müller, P. Vegan Diet in Young Children. *Nestle Nutrition Institute workshop series* **93,** 103–110; 10.1159/000503348 (2020).
10. Yen, C.-E., Yen, C.-H., Huang, M.-C., Cheng, C.-H. & Huang, Y.-C. Dietary intake and nutritional status of vegetarian and omnivorous preschool children and their parents in Taiwan. *Nutrition research (New York, N.Y.)* **28,** 430–436; 10.1016/j.nutres.2008.03.012 (2008).
11. Ambroszkiewicz, J. *et al.* Bone status and adipokine levels in children on vegetarian and omnivorous diets. *Clinical nutrition (Edinburgh, Scotland)* **38,** 730–737; 10.1016/j.clnu.2018.03.010 (2019).
12. Alvisi, P. *et al.* Recommendations on complementary feeding for healthy, full-term infants. *Italian journal of pediatrics* **41,** 36; 10.1186/s13052-015-0143-5 (2015).
13. Thorisdottir, B. *et al.* Infant Feeding, Vitamin D and IgE Sensitization to Food Allergens at 6 Years in a Longitudinal Icelandic Cohort. *Nutrients* **11**; 10.3390/nu11071690 (2019).

14. Kılınç, S., Atay, E., Ceran, Ö. & Atay, Z. Evaluation of vitamin D status and its correlation with gonadal function in children at mini-puberty. *Clinical endocrinology*; 10.1111/cen.13856 (2018).

15. Chen, C.-M. *et al.* Infants' Vitamin D Nutritional Status in the First Year of Life in Northern Taiwan. *Nutrients* **12**; 10.3390/nu12020404 (2020).

16. Andersson, M. *et al.* The Swiss iodized salt program provides adequate iodine for school children and pregnant women, but weaning infants not receiving iodine-containing complementary foods as well as their mothers are iodine deficient. *The Journal of clinical endocrinology and metabolism* **95,** 5217–5224; 10.1210/jc.2010-0975 (2010).

17. Menal-Puey, S., Martínez-Biarge, M. & Marques-Lopes, I. Developing a Food Exchange System for Meal Planning in Vegan Children and Adolescents. *Nutrients* **11**; 10.3390/nu11010043 (2018).

18. Yeliosof, O. & Silverman, L. A. Veganism as a cause of iodine deficient hypothyroidism. *Journal of pediatric endocrinology & metabolism : JPEM* **31,** 91–94; 10.1515/jpem-2017-0082 (2018).

19. Melina, V., Craig, W. & Levin, S. Position of the Academy of Nutrition and Dietetics: vegetarian diets. *Journal of the Academy of Nutrition and Dietetics* **116,** 1970–1980; 10.1016/j.jand.2016.09.025 (2016).

20. Mangels, A. R. & Messina, V. Considerations in planning vegan diets: infants. *Journal of the American Dietetic Association* **101,** 670–677; 10.1016/S0002-8223(01)00169-9 (2001).

21. Palacios, A. M. *et al.* Zinc deficiency associated with anaemia among young children in rural Guatemala. *Maternal & child nutrition* **16,** e12885; 10.1111/mcn.12885 (2020).

22. Zhu, Z. *et al.* Association of infant and young child feeding practices with cognitive development at 10-12 years: A birth cohort in rural western China. *The British journal of nutrition,* 1–32; 10.1017/S0007114519003271 (2019).

23. Santos, H. O., Teixeira, F. J. & Schoenfeld, B. J. Dietary vs. pharmacological doses of zinc: A clinical review. *Clinical nutrition (Edinburgh, Scotland)*; 10.1016/j.clnu.2019.06.024 (2019).

24. Liu, E. *et al.* Effect of Zinc Supplementation on Growth Outcomes in Children under 5 Years of Age. *Nutrients* **10**; 10.3390/nu10030377 (2018).

25. Ackland, M. L. & Michalczyk, A. A. Zinc and infant nutrition. *Archives of biochemistry and biophysics* **611,** 51–57; 10.1016/j.abb.2016.06.011 (2016).

26. He, M.-J., Zhang, S.-Q., Mu, W. & Huang, Z.-W. Selenium in infant formula milk. *Asia Pacific journal of clinical nutrition* **27,** 284–292; 10.6133/apjcn.042017.12 (2018).

27. Zemrani, B., McCallum, Z. & Bines, J. E. Trace Element Provision in Parenteral Nutrition in Children: One Size Does Not Fit All. *Nutrients* **10**; 10.3390/nu10111819 (2018).

34

28. Lönnerdal, B., Vargas-Fernández, E. & Whitacre, M. Selenium fortification of infant formulas: does selenium form matter? *Food & function* **8**, 3856–3868; 10.1039/c7fo00746a (2017).

29. Jin, Y., Coad, J., Weber, J. L., Thomson, J. S. & Brough, L. Selenium Intake in Iodine-Deficient Pregnant and Breastfeeding Women in New Zealand. *Nutrients* **11**; 10.3390/nu11010069 (2019).

30. Fábelová, L. *et al.* Hair concentration of trace elements and growth in homeless children aged <6years: Results from the ENFAMS study. *Environment international* **114**, 318–325; 10.1016/j.envint.2017.10.012 (2018).

31. Iannotti, L. *et al.* Egg intervention effect on linear growth no longer present after two years. *Maternal & child nutrition,* e12925; 10.1111/mcn.12925 (2019).

32. Warren, J. An update on complementary feeding. *Nursing children and young people* **30**, 38–47; 10.7748/ncyp.2018.e1032 (2018).

33. Henjum, S. *et al.* Suboptimal Iodine Concentration in Breastmilk and Inadequate Iodine Intake among Lactating Women in Norway. *Nutrients* **9**; 10.3390/nu9070643 (2017).

34. Pawlak, R. To vegan or not to vegan when pregnant, lactating or feeding young children. *European journal of clinical nutrition*; 10.1038/ejcn.2017.111 (2017).

35. Zielinska, M. A., Hamulka, J., Grabowicz-Chądrzyńska, I., Bryś, J. & Wesolowska, A. Association between Breastmilk LC PUFA, Carotenoids and Psychomotor Development of Exclusively Breastfed Infants. *International journal of environmental research and public health* **16**; 10.3390/ijerph16071144 (2019).

36. Karcz, K. & Królak-Olejnik, B. Vegan or vegetarian diet and breast milk composition - a systematic review. *Critical reviews in food science and nutrition,* 1–18; 10.1080/10408398.2020.1753650 (2020).

37. Eidelman, A. I. Exclusive Breastfeeding and Complementary Feedings Are Not Mutually Exclusive. *Breastfeeding medicine : the official journal of the Academy of Breastfeeding Medicine* **13**, 93–94; 10.1089/bfm.2018.29067.aie (2018).

38. Houghton, L. A. *et al.* Micronutrient status differs among Maasai and Kamba preschoolers in a supplementary feeding programme in Kenya. *Maternal & child nutrition* **15**, e12805; 10.1111/mcn.12805 (2019).

39. Netting, M. J. & Makrides, M. Complementary Foods: Guidelines and Practices. *Nestle Nutrition Institute workshop series* **87**, 1–12; 10.1159/000449497 (2017).

40. West, C. Introduction of Complementary Foods to Infants. *Annals of nutrition & metabolism* **70 Suppl 2,** 47–54; 10.1159/000457928 (2017).

41. Phillips, J. T., Stahlhut, R. W., Looney, R. J. & Järvinen, K. M. Food Allergy, Breastfeeding and Introduction of Complementary Foods in the New York Old Order Mennonites. *Annals of allergy, asthma & immunology : official publication of the American College of Allergy, Asthma, & Immunology*; 10.1016/j.anai.2019.12.019 (2020).

42. Ahmed, K. Y., Page, A., Arora, A. & Ogbo, F. A. Trends and factors associated with complementary feeding practices in Ethiopia from 2005 to 2016. *Maternal & child nutrition,* e12926; 10.1111/mcn.12926 (2019).

43. Papanikolaou, Y. & Fulgoni, V. L. Grain Foods in US Infants Are Associated with Greater Nutrient Intakes, Improved Diet Quality and Increased Consumption of Recommended Food Groups. *Nutrients* **11**; 10.3390/nu11122840 (2019).

44. Smith, J. D. *et al.* Association between Ready-to-Eat Cereal Consumption and Nutrient Intake, Nutritional Adequacy, and Diet Quality among Infants, Toddlers, and Children in the National Health and Nutrition Examination Survey 2015-2016. *Nutrients* **11**; 10.3390/nu11091989 (2019).

45. Baroni, L. *et al.* Vegan Nutrition for Mothers and Children: Practical Tools for Healthcare Providers. *Nutrients* **11**; 10.3390/nu11010005 (2018).

46. Baroni, L., Goggi, S. & Battino, M. Planning Well-Balanced Vegetarian Diets in Infants, Children, and Adolescents. The VegPlate Junior. *Journal of the Academy of Nutrition and Dietetics*; 10.1016/j.jand.2018.06.008 (2019).

47. Khamis, A. G., Mwanri, A. W., Ntwenya, J. E. & Kreppel, K. The influence of dietary diversity on the nutritional status of children between 6 and 23 months of age in Tanzania. *BMC pediatrics* **19,** 518; 10.1186/s12887-019-1897-5 (2019).

48. Wikström, S. & Holst, E. Spädbarnsbotulism – skäl att inte ge honung till barn under ett år. *Lakartidningen* **114** (2017).

49. Grabowski, N. T. & Klein, G. Microbiology and foodborne pathogens in honey. *Critical reviews in food science and nutrition* **57,** 1852–1862; 10.1080/10408398.2015.1029041 (2017).

50. Paccione, R., Remedios, P., Gautreaux, J. & English, R. Diffuse Muscle Weakness in an Infant. *Clinical pediatrics* **54,** 1394–1395; 10.1177/0009922815570626 (2015).

51. PAHO & WHO. Guiding principles for complementary feeding of the breastfed child. Available at https://www.who.int/maternal_child_adolescent/documents/a85622/en/ (2003).

52. WHO. Why can't we give water to a breastfeeding baby before the 6 months, even when it is hot? Available at https://www.who.int/news-room/q-a-detail/why-can-t-we-give-water-to-a-breastfeeding-baby-before-the-6-months-even-when-it-is-hot# (2020).

53. Levine Obe, R. S. Might one simple question indicate a child's caries risk and guide preventive advice? *British dental journal* **227,** 834–836; 10.1038/s41415-019-0858-6 (2019).

54. Porter, R. M. *et al.* A Review of Modifiable Risk Factors for Severe Obesity in Children Ages 5 and Under. *Childhood obesity (Print)* **14,** 468–476; 10.1089/chi.2017.0344 (2018).

55. Kim, H.-Y. *et al.* Prolonged bedtime bottle feeding and respiratory symptoms in infants. *Asia Pacific allergy* **1,** 30–35; 10.5415/apallergy.2011.1.1.30 (2011).

56. Brambilla, P. *et al.* Sleep habits and pattern in 1-14 years old children and relationship with video devices use and evening and night child activities. *Italian journal of pediatrics* **43,** 7; 10.1186/s13052-016-0324-x (2017).

57. Brecher, E. A. & Lewis, C. W. Infant Oral Health. *Pediatric clinics of North America* **65,** 909–921; 10.1016/j.pcl.2018.05.016 (2018).

58. Siauw, C., Wirbelauer, J., Schweitzer, T. & Speer, C. P. Late Vitamin K Deficient Bleeding in 2 Young Infants--Renaissance of a Preventable Disease. *Zeitschrift fur Geburtshilfe und Neonatologie* **219,** 238–242; 10.1055/s-0035-1555873 (2015).

59. Kühnisch, J. *et al.* Fluoride/vitamin D tablet supplementation in infants-effects on dental health after 10 years. *Clinical oral investigations* **21,** 2283–2290; 10.1007/s00784-016-2021-y (2017).

60. Wagner, Y. & Heinrich-Weltzien, R. Evaluation of an interdisciplinary preventive programme for early childhood caries: findings of a regional German birth cohort study. *Clinical oral investigations* **20,** 1943–1952; 10.1007/s00784-015-1685-z (2016).

61. Zohoori, F. V. & Duckworth, R. M. Chapter 5: Microelements: Part II: F, Al, Mo and Co. *Monographs in oral science* **28,** 48–58; 10.1159/000455370 (2020).

62. Lessen, R. & Kavanagh, K. Position of the academy of nutrition and dietetics: promoting and supporting breastfeeding. *Journal of the Academy of Nutrition and Dietetics* **115,** 444–449; 10.1016/j.jand.2014.12.014 (2015).

63. Johnston, M., Landers, S., Noble, L., Szucs, K. & Viehmann, L. Breastfeeding and the use of human milk. *Pediatrics* **129,** e827-41; 10.1542/peds.2011-3552 (2012).

64. SACN. Feeding in the First Year of Life. Published July 2018. Available at https://assets.publishing.service.gov.uk/government/uploads/system/u ploads/attachment_data/file/725530/SACN_report_on_Feeding_in_the _First_Year_of_Life.pdf (2018).

65. Critch, J. N. Nutrition for healthy term infants, six to 24 months: An overview. *Paediatrics & child health* **19,** 547–552 (2014).

66. Canadian Paediatric Society. The use of fluoride in infants and children. *Paediatrics & child health* **7,** 569–582; 10.1093/pch/7.8.569 (2002).

67. Ng, E. & Loewy, A. D. Guidelines for vitamin K prophylaxis in newborns. *Paediatrics & child health* **23,** 394–402; 10.1093/pch/pxy082 (2018).

68. Bouillon, R. Comparative analysis of nutritional guidelines for vitamin D. *Nature reviews. Endocrinology* **13,** 466–479; 10.1038/nrendo.2017.31 (2017).

69. Uday, S., Kongjonaj, A., Aguiar, M., Tulchinsky, T. & Högler, W. Variations in infant and childhood vitamin D supplementation programmes across Europe and factors influencing adherence. *Endocrine connections* **6,** 667–675; 10.1530/EC-17-0193 (2017).

70. Mihatsch, W. A. *et al.* Prevention of Vitamin K Deficiency Bleeding in Newborn Infants: A Position Paper by the ESPGHAN Committee on Nutrition. *Journal of pediatric gastroenterology and nutrition* **63,** 123–129; 10.1097/MPG.0000000000001232 (2016).

71. Prell, C. & Koletzko, B. Breastfeeding and Complementary Feeding. *Deutsches Arzteblatt international* **113,** 435–444; 10.3238/arztebl.2016.0435 (2016).

72. Strehle, E.-M., Howey, C. & Jones, R. Evaluation of the acceptability of a new oral vitamin K prophylaxis for breastfed infants. *Acta paediatrica (Oslo, Norway : 1992)* **99,** 379–383; 10.1111/j.1651-2227.2009.01630.x (2010).

73. Waheed, N. *et al.* Vitamin D Intoxication In 7-Month-Old Infant With Recommended Daily Intake Of Vitamin D. *Journal of Ayub Medical College, Abbottabad : JAMC* **30(Suppl 1),** S673-S675 (2018).

74. Pludowski, P. *et al.* Vitamin D supplementation guidelines. *The Journal of steroid biochemistry and molecular biology* **175,** 125–135; 10.1016/j.jsbmb.2017.01.021 (2018).

75. Ross, A. C., Taylor, C. L., Yaktine, A. L. & Cook, H. D. (eds.). *Dietary Reference Intakes for Calcium and Vitamin D* (National Academies Press, Washington, DC, 2011).

76. BNF. Nutrition Requirements. Available at https://www.nutrition.org.uk/attachments/article/234/Nutrition%20Re quirements_Revised%20Oct%202016.pdf (2016).

77. Priyadarshi, M. *et al.* Efficacy of daily supplementation of 800 IU vitamin D on vitamin D status at 6 months of age in term healthy Indian infants. *Journal of perinatology : official journal of the California Perinatal Association*; 10.1038/s41372-018-0216-6 (2018).

78. NIH. Vitamin D Fact Sheet for Health Professionals. Available at https://ods.od.nih.gov/factsheets/VitaminD-HealthProfessional/ (2020).

79. IOM, Ross, A. C., Taylor, C. L. & Yaktine, A. L. *Dietary reference intakes for calcium and vitamin D* (National Academies Press, Washington, DC, 2011).

80. Marra, M. V. & Bailey, R. L. Position of the Academy of Nutrition and Dietetics: Micronutrient Supplementation. *Journal of the Academy of Nutrition and Dietetics* **118,** 2162–2173; 10.1016/j.jand.2018.07.022 (2018).

81. BNF. SACN's 'Feeding in the First Year of Life' report published. Available at https://www.nutrition.org.uk/nutritioninthenews/new-reports/feedinginthefirstyear.html (2018).

82. Crawley, H. *Eating well. Vegan infants and under-5s* (First Steps Nutrition Trust, 2017).

83. BDA. Complementary feeding (weaning): Food Fact Sheet. Available at https://www.bda.uk.com/resource/complementary-feeding-weaning.html (2019).

84. Robinson, S. L., Ramirez-Zea, M., Roman, A. V. & Villamor, E. Correlates and family aggregation of vitamin D concentrations in school-aged children and their parents in nine Mesoamerican countries. *Public health nutrition,* 1–12; 10.1017/S1368980017001616 (2017).

85. Chang, S.-W. & Lee, H.-C. Vitamin D and health - The missing vitamin in humans. *Pediatrics and neonatology* **60,** 237–244; 10.1016/j.pedneo.2019.04.007 (2019).

86. Jindal, A. K., Gupta, A., Vinay, K. & Bishnoi, A. Sun Exposure in Children: Balancing the Benefits and Harms. *Indian dermatology online journal* **11,** 94–98; 10.4103/idoj.IDOJ_206_19 (2020).

87. Magalhaes, S. *et al.* Shedding light on the link between early life sun exposure and risk of multiple sclerosis: results from the EnvIMS Study. *International journal of epidemiology* **48,** 1073–1082; 10.1093/ije/dyy269 (2019).

88. Rueter, K. *et al.* Direct infant UV light exposure is associated with eczema and immune development. *The Journal of allergy and clinical immunology* **143,** 1012-1020.e2; 10.1016/j.jaci.2018.08.037 (2019).

89. Matsushima, Y., Mizutani, K., Yamaguchi, Y. & Yamanaka, K. Vitamin D is no substitute for the sun. *The Journal of allergy and clinical immunology*; 10.1016/j.jaci.2019.01.004 (2019).

90. Di Marco, N., Kaufman, J. & Rodda, C. P. Shedding Light on Vitamin D Status and Its Complexities during Pregnancy, Infancy and Childhood: An Australian Perspective. *International journal of environmental research and public health* **16**; 10.3390/ijerph16040538 (2019).

91. Antonucci, R., Locci, C., Clemente, M. G., Chicconi, E. & Antonucci, L. Vitamin D deficiency in childhood: old lessons and current challenges. *Journal of pediatric endocrinology & metabolism : JPEM* **31,** 247–260; 10.1515/jpem-2017-0391 (2018).

92. AAPD. Fluoride Therapy. Latest Revision 2018. *The Reference Manual of Pediatric Dentistry,* 262–265 (2018).

93. CDA. CDA Position on Use of Fluorides in Caries Prevention. This statement is currently under the Canadian Dental Association review process. Available at https://www.cda-adc.ca/en/about/position_statements/fluoride/ (2020).

94. Harriehausen, C. X., Dosani, F. Z., Chiquet, B. T., Barratt, M. S. & Quock, R. L. Fluoride Intake of Infants from Formula. *The Journal of clinical pediatric dentistry* **43,** 34–41; 10.17796/1053-4625-43.1.7 (2019).

95. Zohoori, F. V., Omid, N., Sanderson, R. A., Valentine, R. A. & Maguire, A. Fluoride retention in infants living in fluoridated and non-fluoridated areas: effects of weaning. *The British journal of nutrition* **121,** 74–81; 10.1017/S0007114518003008 (2019).

96. Whelton, H. P., Spencer, A. J., Do, L. G. & Rugg-Gunn, A. J. Fluoride Revolution and Dental Caries: Evolution of Policies for Global Use. *Journal of dental research* **98,** 837–846; 10.1177/0022034519843495 (2019).

97. Till, C. *et al.* Fluoride exposure from infant formula and child IQ in a Canadian birth cohort. *Environment international* **134,** 105315; 10.1016/j.envint.2019.105315 (2020).

98. Devenish, G. *et al.* Early childhood feeding practices and dental caries among Australian preschoolers. *The American journal of clinical nutrition*; 10.1093/ajcn/nqaa012 (2020).

99. Wagner, Y. & Heinrich-Weltzien, R. Risk factors for dental problems: Recommendations for oral health in infancy. *Early human development* **114,** 16–21; 10.1016/j.earlhumdev.2017.09.009 (2017).

100. Wright, J. T. *et al.* Fluoride toothpaste efficacy and safety in children younger than 6 years: a systematic review. *Journal of the American Dental Association (1939)* **145,** 182–189; 10.14219/jada.2013.37 (2014).

101. AAP. Working Together: Breastfeeding and Solid Foods. Source: Adapted from New Mother's Guide to Breastfeeding, 2nd Edition (Copyright © 2011 American Academy of Pediatrics). Available at https://www.healthychildren.org/English/ages-stages/baby/breastfeeding/Pages/Working-Together-Breastfeeding-and-Solid-Foods.aspx (2020).

102. Baker, R. D. & Greer, F. R. Diagnosis and prevention of iron deficiency and iron-deficiency anemia in infants and young children (0-3 years of age). *Pediatrics* **126,** 1040–1050; 10.1542/peds.2010-2576 (2010).

103. Paganini, D. & Zimmermann, M. B. The effects of iron fortification and supplementation on the gut microbiome and diarrhea in infants and children: a review. *The American journal of clinical nutrition* **106,** 1688S–1693S; 10.3945/ajcn.117.156067 (2017).

104. Suchdev, P. S., Jefferds, M. E. D., Ota, E., da Silva Lopes, K. & De-Regil, L. M. Home fortification of foods with multiple micronutrient powders for health and nutrition in children under two years of age. *The Cochrane database of systematic reviews* **2,** CD008959; 10.1002/14651858.CD008959.pub3 (2020).

105. Campos Ponce, M. *et al.* What Approaches are Most Effective at Addressing Micronutrient Deficiency in Children 0-5 Years? A Review of Systematic Reviews. *Maternal and child health journal* **23**, 4–17; 10.1007/s10995-018-2527-9 (2019).

106. Cusick, S. E., Georgieff, M. K. & Rao, R. Approaches for Reducing the Risk of Early-Life Iron Deficiency-Induced Brain Dysfunction in Children. *Nutrients* **10**; 10.3390/nu10020227 (2018).

107. Agnoli, C. *et al.* Position paper on vegetarian diets from the working group of the Italian Society of Human Nutrition. *Nutrition, metabolism, and cardiovascular diseases : NMCD* **27**, 1037–1052; 10.1016/j.numecd.2017.10.020 (2017).

108. Lönnerdal, B. Development of iron homeostasis in infants and young children. *The American journal of clinical nutrition* **106**, 1575S-1580S; 10.3945/ajcn.117.155820 (2017).

109. Gozzelino, R. & Arosio, P. Iron Homeostasis in Health and Disease. *International journal of molecular sciences* **17**; 10.3390/ijms17010130 (2016).

110. Lönnerdal, B. Excess iron intake as a factor in growth, infections, and development of infants and young children. *The American journal of clinical nutrition* **106**, 1681S-1687S; 10.3945/ajcn.117.156042 (2017).

111. Cox, K. A. *et al.* Association Between Meat and Meat-Alternative Consumption and Iron Stores in Early Childhood. *Academic pediatrics* **16**, 783–791; 10.1016/j.acap.2016.01.003 (2016).

112. Jager, I. de, Borgonjen-van den Berg, K. J., Giller, K. E. & Brouwer, I. D. Current and potential role of grain legumes on protein and micronutrient adequacy of the diet of rural Ghanaian infants and young children: using linear programming. *Nutrition journal* **18**, 12; 10.1186/s12937-019-0435-5 (2019).

113. Ferguson, E., Chege, P., Kimiywe, J., Wiesmann, D. & Hotz, C. Zinc, iron and calcium are major limiting nutrients in the complementary diets of rural Kenyan children. *Maternal & child nutrition* **11 Suppl 3**, 6–20; 10.1111/mcn.12243 (2015).

114. Lemoine, A., Giabicani, E., Lockhart, V., Grimprel, E. & Tounian, P. Case report of nutritional rickets in an infant following a vegan diet. *Archives de pediatrie : organe officiel de la Societe francaise de pediatrie*; 10.1016/j.arcped.2020.03.008 (2020).

115. Tandoi, F., Morlacchi, L., Bossi, A. & Agosti, M. Introducing complementary foods in the first year of life. *La Pediatria medica e chirurgica : Medical and surgical pediatrics* **39**, 186; 10.4081/pmc.2017.186 (2017).

116. Romero-Velarde, E. *et al.* Consenso para las prácticas de alimentación complementaria en lactantes sanos. *Boletin medico del Hospital Infantil de Mexico* **73**, 338–356; 10.1016/j.bmhimx.2016.06.007 (2016).

117. O'Connell, J. M. *et al.* Growth of vegetarian children: the Farm study. *Pediatrics* **84**, 475–481 (1989).

41

118. Sanders, T. A. & Reddy, S. Vegetarian diets and children. *The American journal of clinical nutrition* **59,** 1176S-1181S (1994).

119. Sanders, T. A. B. & Manning, J. The growth and development of vegan children. *J Hum Nutr Diet* **5,** 11–21; 10.1111/j.1365-277X.1992.tb00129.x (1992).

120. Sanders, T. A. Growth and development of British vegan children. *The American journal of clinical nutrition* **48,** 822–825 (1988).

121. Sanders, T. A. & Purves, R. An anthropometric and dietary assessment of the nutritional status of vegan preschool children. Abstract. *Journal of human nutrition* **35,** 349–357 (1981).

122. Weder, S., Hoffmann, M., Becker, K., Alexy, U. & Keller, M. Energy, Macronutrient Intake, and Anthropometrics of Vegetarian, Vegan, and Omnivorous Children (1‾3 Years) in Germany (VeChi Diet Study). *Nutrients* **11**; 10.3390/nu11040832 (2019).

123. Willett, W. *et al.* Food in the Anthropocene: the EAT–Lancet Commission on healthy diets from sustainable food systems. *The Lancet* **393,** 447–492; 10.1016/S0140-6736(18)31788-4 (2019).

124. Were, F. N. & Lifschitz, C. Complementary Feeding: Beyond Nutrition. *Annals of nutrition & metabolism* **73 Suppl 1,** 20–25; 10.1159/000490084 (2018).

125. Phang, M. *et al.* Epigenetic aging in newborns: role of maternal diet. *The American journal of clinical nutrition* **111,** 555–561; 10.1093/ajcn/nqz326 (2020).

126. Redecillas, S., Moráis, A., Marques, I. & Moreno-Villares, J. M. Guía de recomendaciones sobre las dietas vegetarianas en niños. *Anales de pediatria (Barcelona, Spain : 2003)*; 10.1016/j.anpedi.2018.09.012 (2018).

127. IOM. *Institute of Medicine (IOM): Dietary Reference Intakes for Thiamin, Riboflavin, Niacin, Vitamin B6, Folate, Vitamin B12, Pantothenic Acid, Biotin, and Choline* (Washington (DC), 1998).

128. Ströhle, A. *et al.* The Revised D-A-CH-Reference Values for the Intake of Vitamin B12 : Prevention of Deficiency and Beyond. *Molecular nutrition & food research* **63,** e1801178; 10.1002/mnfr.201801178 (2019).

129. Obeid, R. *et al.* Vitamin B12 Intake From Animal Foods, Biomarkers, and Health Aspects. *Frontiers in nutrition* **6,** 93; 10.3389/fnut.2019.00093 (2019).

130. Zimmermann, M. B. The Importance of Adequate Iodine during Pregnancy and Infancy. *World review of nutrition and dietetics* **115,** 118–124; 10.1159/000442078 (2016).

131. Andersson, M., Benoist, B. de, Delange, F. & Zupan, J. Prevention and control of iodine deficiency in pregnant and lactating women and in children less than 2-years-old: conclusions and recommendations of the Technical Consultation. *Public health nutrition* **10,** 1606–1611; 10.1017/S1368980007361004 (2007).

132. Dold, S. *et al.* Universal Salt Iodization Provides Sufficient Dietary Iodine to Achieve Adequate Iodine Nutrition during the First 1000 Days: A Cross-Sectional Multicenter Study. *The Journal of nutrition* **148,** 587–598; 10.1093/jn/nxy015 (2018).

133. World Health Organization (WHO). *Assessment of iodine deficiency disorders and monitoring their elimination. A guide for programme managers.* 3rd ed. (World Health Organization, Geneva, 2007).

134. Dumrongwongsiri, O. *et al.* High Urinary Iodine Concentration Among Breastfed Infants and the Factors Associated with Iodine Content in Breast Milk. *Biological trace element research* **186,** 106–113; 10.1007/s12011-018-1303-4 (2018).

135. Jorgensen, A., O'Leary, P., James, I., Skeaff, S. & Sherriff, J. Assessment of Breast Milk Iodine Concentrations in Lactating Women in Western Australia. *Nutrients* **8**; 10.3390/nu8110699 (2016).

136. Hwang, E.-S., Ki, K.-N. & Chung, H.-Y. Proximate composition, amino Acid, mineral, and heavy metal content of dried laver. *Preventive nutrition and food science* **18,** 139–144; 10.3746/pnf.2013.18.2.139 (2013).

137. Kawasaki, A. *et al.* The Taurine Content of Japanese Seaweed. *Advances in experimental medicine and biology* **975 Pt 2,** 1105–1112; 10.1007/978-94-024-1079-2_88 (2017).

138. Ross, A. C., Taylor, C. L., Yaktine, A. L. & Del Valle, H. B. (eds.). *Dietary Reference Intakes for Calcium and Vitamin D* (Washington (DC), 2011).

139. Turck, D. *et al.* Update of the tolerable upper intake level for vitamin D for infants. *EFS2* **16**; 10.2903/j.efsa.2018.5365 (2018).

140. Kocaoglu, C. *et al.* Cerebral atrophy in a vitamin B12-deficient infant of a vegetarian mother. *Journal of health, population, and nutrition* **32,** 367–371 (2014).

141. Vats, P., Verma, P., Varughese, B., Kumar, S. & Kapoor, S. Frontotemporal Atrophy. Presenting Sign in Infantile Cobalamin Deficiency. *Indian journal of pediatrics*; 10.1007/s12098-017-2542-7 (2017).

142. Priyankara, W. D. D., Chandimal, A. V. I., Sivagnanam, F. G. & Manoj, E. M. Cerebral Venous Sinus Thrombosis and Hydrocephalus in a Vegan Secondary to Acquired Hyperhomocystinaemia. *Case Reports in Critical Care* **2019**; 10.1155/2019/1468704 (2019).

143. Wighton, M. C., Manson, J. I., Speed, I., Robertson, E. & Chapman, E. BRAIN DAMAGE IN INFANCY AND DIETARY VITAMIN B 12 DEFICIENCY. *Med J Aust* **2,** 1–3; 10.5694/j.1326-5377.1979.tb112643.x (1979).

144. Bettinelli, M. E. *et al.* Knowledge of Health Professionals Regarding Vegetarian Diets from Pregnancy to Adolescence: An Observational Study. *Nutrients* **11**; 10.3390/nu11051149 (2019).

145. Gramer, G. *et al.* Newborn Screening for Vitamin B12 Deficiency in Germany-Strategies, Results, and Public Health Implications. *The Journal of pediatrics*; 10.1016/j.jpeds.2019.07.052 (2019).

43

146. Pawlak, R. *et al.* Vitamin B-12 content in breast milk of vegan, vegetarian, and nonvegetarian lactating women in the United States. *The American journal of clinical nutrition*; 10.1093/ajcn/nqy104 (2018).

147. Amorós, R. *et al.* Maternal selenium status and neuropsychological development in Spanish preschool children. *Environmental research* **166,** 215–222; 10.1016/j.envres.2018.06.002 (2018).

148. Li, C., Solomons, N. W., Scott, M. E. & Koski, K. G. Minerals and Trace Elements in Human Breast Milk Are Associated with Guatemalan Infant Anthropometric Outcomes within the First 6 Months. *The Journal of nutrition* **146,** 2067–2074; 10.3945/jn.116.232223 (2016).

149. Sebastiani, G. *et al.* The Effects of Vegetarian and Vegan Diet during Pregnancy on the Health of Mothers and Offspring. *Nutrients* **11**; 10.3390/nu11030557 (2019).

150. Reynolds, A., O'Connell, S. M., Kenny, L. C. & Dempsey, E. Transient neonatal hypercalcaemia secondary to excess maternal vitamin D intake: too much of a good thing. *BMJ case reports* **2017**; 10.1136/bcr-2016-219043 (2017).

151. Hollis, B. W. *et al.* Maternal Versus Infant Vitamin D Supplementation During Lactation: A Randomized Controlled Trial. *Pediatrics* **136,** 625–634; 10.1542/peds.2015-1669 (2015).

152. Eastman, C. J., Ma, G. & Li, M. Optimal Assessment and Quantification of Iodine Nutrition in Pregnancy and Lactation: Laboratory and Clinical Methods, Controversies and Future Directions. *Nutrients* **11**; 10.3390/nu11102378 (2019).

153. Burdge, G. C., Tan, S.-Y. & Henry, C. J. Long-chain n-3 PUFA in vegetarian women: a metabolic perspective. *Journal of nutritional science* **6,** e58; 10.1017/jns.2017.62 (2017).

154. Sanders, T. A., Ellis, F. R. & Dickerson, J. W. Studies of vegans: the fatty acid composition of plasma choline phosphoglycerides, erythrocytes, adipose tissue, and breast milk, and some indicators of susceptibility to ischemic heart disease in vegans and omnivore controls. *The American journal of clinical nutrition* **31,** 805–813; 10.1093/ajcn/31.5.805 (1978).

155. Dinh, Q. T. *et al.* Selenium distribution in the Chinese environment and its relationship with human health. A review. *Environment international* **112,** 294–309; 10.1016/j.envint.2017.12.035 (2018).

156. Combs, G. F. Selenium in global food systems. *The British journal of nutrition* **85,** 517–547 (2001).

157. Kipp, A. P. *et al.* Revised reference values for selenium intake. *Journal of trace elements in medicine and biology : organ of the Society for Minerals and Trace Elements (GMS)* **32,** 195–199; 10.1016/j.jtemb.2015.07.005 (2015).

158. Yu, K. *et al.* Translation of nutrient recommendations into personalized optimal diets for Chinese urban lactating women by linear programming models. *BMC pregnancy and childbirth* **18,** 379; 10.1186/s12884-018-2008-6 (2018).

159. IOM. *Dietary reference intakes for vitamin C, vitamin E, selenium, and carotenoids. A report of the Panel on Dietary Antioxidants and Related Compounds, Subcommittees on Upper Reference Levels of Nutrients and of Interpretation and Use of Dietary Reference Intakes, and the Standing Committee on the Scientific Evaluation of Dietary Reference Intakes, Food and Nutrition Board, Institute of Medicine* (National Academy Press, Washington, D.C, 2000).

160. Mazokopakis, E. E. & Liontiris, M. I. Commentary. Health Concerns of Brazil Nut Consumption. *Journal of alternative and complementary medicine (New York, N.Y.)* **24,** 3–6; 10.1089/acm.2017.0159 (2018).

161. Donadio, J. L. S. *et al.* Genetic variants in selenoprotein genes modulate biomarkers of selenium status in response to Brazil nut supplementation (the SU.BRA.NUT study). *Clinical nutrition (Edinburgh, Scotland)*; 10.1016/j.clnu.2018.03.011 (2018).

162. Henjum, S. *et al.* Vitamin B12 concentrations in milk from Norwegian women during the six first months of lactation. *European journal of clinical nutrition*; 10.1038/s41430-020-0567-x (2020).

163. Steffey, C. L. Pediatric Osteoporosis. *Pediatrics in review* **40,** 259–261; 10.1542/pir.2017-0277 (2019).

164. Chen, C.-M. *et al.* Iron Status of Infants in the First Year of Life in Northern Taiwan. *Nutrients* **12**; 10.3390/nu12010139 (2020).

165. Awasthi, S. *et al.* Micronutrient-fortified infant cereal improves hemoglobin status and reduces iron deficiency anemia in Indian infants: An effectiveness study. *The British journal of nutrition,* 1–26; 10.1017/S0007114519003386 (2020).

166. Lifschitz, C. H. *et al.* Practices of Introduction of Complementary Feeding and Iron Deficiency Prevention in the Middle East and North Africa. *Journal of pediatric gastroenterology and nutrition* **67,** 538–542; 10.1097/MPG.0000000000002059 (2018).

167. He, M.-J. *et al.* Breast milk selenocystine as a biomarker for selenium intake in lactating women at differential geographical deficiency risk in China. *Asia Pacific journal of clinical nutrition* **28,** 341–346; 10.6133/apjcn.201906_28(2).0016 (2019).

168. Sabatier, M. *et al.* Longitudinal Changes of Mineral Concentrations in Preterm and Term Human Milk from Lactating Swiss Women. *Nutrients* **11**; 10.3390/nu11081855 (2019).

169. Daniels, L. *et al.* Micronutrient intakes of lactating mothers and their association with breast milk concentrations and micronutrient adequacy of exclusively breastfed Indonesian infants. *The American journal of clinical nutrition* **110,** 391–400; 10.1093/ajcn/nqz047 (2019).

170. Alves Peixoto, R. R. *et al.* Trace mineral composition of human breast milk from Brazilian mothers. *Journal of trace elements in medicine and biology : organ of the Society for Minerals and Trace Elements (GMS)* **54,** 199–205; 10.1016/j.jtemb.2019.05.002 (2019).

171. Snoj Tratnik, J. *et al.* Results of the first national human biomonitoring in Slovenia: Trace elements in men and lactating women, predictors of exposure and reference values. *International journal of hygiene and environmental health* **222,** 563–582; 10.1016/j.ijheh.2019.02.008 (2019).

172. Valent, F., Horvat, M., Mazej, D., Stibilj, V. & Barbone, F. Maternal diet and selenium concentration in human milk from an Italian population. *Journal of epidemiology* **21,** 285–292; 10.2188/jea.je20100183 (2011).

173. Han, F. *et al.* Calculation of an Adequate Intake (AI) Value and Safe Range of Selenium (Se) for Chinese Infants 0-3 Months Old Based on Se Concentration in the Milk of Lactating Chinese Women with Optimal Se Intake. *Biological trace element research* **188,** 363–372; 10.1007/s12011-018-1440-9 (2019).

174. Dodge, M. L., Wander, R. C., Xia, Y., Butler, J. A. & Whanger, P. D. Glutathione Peroxidase Activity Modulates Fatty Acid Profiles of Plasma and Breast Milk in Chinese Women. *Journal of Trace Elements in Medicine and Biology* **12,** 221–230; 10.1016/S0946-672X(99)80062-5 (1999).

175. Dorea, J. G. Selenium and breast-feeding. *The British journal of nutrition* **88,** 443–461; 10.1079/BJN2002692 (2002).

176. Hannan, M. A., Faraji, B., Tanguma, J., Longoria, N. & Rodriguez, R. C. Maternal milk concentration of zinc, iron, selenium, and iodine and its relationship to dietary intakes. *Biological trace element research* **127,** 6–15; 10.1007/s12011-008-8221-9 (2009).

177. Gu, Z., Silva, S. de & Reichman, S. M. Arsenic Concentrations and Dietary Exposure in Rice-Based Infant Food in Australia. *International journal of environmental research and public health* **17**; 10.3390/ijerph17020415 (2020).

178. Iannotti, L. L. *et al.* Eggs early in complementary feeding increase choline pathway biomarkers and DHA: a randomized controlled trial in Ecuador. *The American journal of clinical nutrition* **106,** 1482–1489; 10.3945/ajcn.117.160515 (2017).

179. Wallace, T. C. *et al.* Choline: The Underconsumed and Underappreciated Essential Nutrient. *Nutrition today* **53,** 240–253; 10.1097/NT.0000000000000302 (2018).

180. Signes-Pastor, A. J. *et al.* Levels of infants' urinary arsenic metabolites related to formula feeding and weaning with rice products exceeding the EU inorganic arsenic standard. *PloS one* **12,** e0176923; 10.1371/journal.pone.0176923 (2017).

181. Guillod-Magnin, R., Brüschweiler, B. J., Aubert, R. & Haldimann, M. Arsenic species in rice and rice-based products consumed by toddlers in Switzerland. *Food additives & contaminants. Part A, Chemistry, analysis, control, exposure & risk assessment* **35,** 1164–1178; 10.1080/19440049.2018.1440641 (2018).

182. Carignan, C. C., Punshon, T., Karagas, M. R. & Cottingham, K. L. Potential Exposure to Arsenic from Infant Rice Cereal. *Annals of global health* **82,** 221–224; 10.1016/j.aogh.2016.01.020 (2016).

183. Jackson, B. P., Taylor, V. F., Karagas, M. R., Punshon, T. & Cottingham, K. L. Arsenic, organic foods, and brown rice syrup. *Environmental health perspectives* **120,** 623–626; 10.1289/ehp.1104619 (2012).

184. Shibata, T., Meng, C., Umoren, J. & West, H. Risk Assessment of Arsenic in Rice Cereal and Other Dietary Sources for Infants and Toddlers in the U.S. *International journal of environmental research and public health* **13,** 361; 10.3390/ijerph13040361 (2016).

185. Signes-Pastor, A. J. *et al.* Infants' dietary arsenic exposure during transition to solid food. *Scientific reports* **8,** 7114; 10.1038/s41598-018-25372-1 (2018).

186. Meyer, R., Carey, M. P., Turner, P. J. & Meharg, A. A. Low inorganic arsenic in hydrolysed rice formula used for cow's milk protein allergy. *Pediatric allergy and immunology : official publication of the European Society of Pediatric Allergy and Immunology* **29,** 561–563; 10.1111/pai.12913 (2018).

187. Chajduk, E., Pyszynska, M. & Polkowska-Motrenko, H. Determination of Trace Elements in Infant Formulas Available on Polish Market. *Biological trace element research* **186,** 589–596; 10.1007/s12011-018-1339-5 (2018).

188. Choi, J. *et al.* Low-Level Toxic Metal Exposure in Healthy Weaning-Age Infants: Association with Growth, Dietary Intake, and Iron Deficiency. *International journal of environmental research and public health* **14**; 10.3390/ijerph14040388 (2017).

189. Rippey, P. L. F., Aravena, F. & Nyonator, J. P. Health Impacts of Early Complementary Food Introduction between Formula-Fed and Breastfed Infants. *Journal of pediatric gastroenterology and nutrition*; 10.1097/MPG.0000000000002581 (2019).

190. Smith, H. A. & Becker, G. E. Early additional food and fluids for healthy breastfed full-term infants. *The Cochrane database of systematic reviews,* CD006462; 10.1002/14651858.CD006462.pub4 (2016).

191. Eidelman, A. I. The Risk of Supplementing Breastfeeding with a Cow's Milk-Based Formula. *Breastfeeding medicine : the official journal of the Academy of Breastfeeding Medicine*; 10.1089/bfm.2019.29146.aie (2020).

192. Mph, J. B. Infant Formula: An Analysis of the Contents of Plant-Based vs. Whey-Based Formulas (P11-056-19). *Current developments in nutrition* **3**; 10.1093/cdn/nzz048.P11-056-19 (2019).

193. Testa, I. *et al.* Soy-Based Infant Formula: Are Phyto-Oestrogens Still in Doubt? *Frontiers in nutrition* **5,** 110; 10.3389/fnut.2018.00110 (2018).

194. Vandenplas, Y. *et al.* Safety of soya-based infant formulas in children. *The British journal of nutrition* **111,** 1340–1360; 10.1017/S0007114513003942 (2014).

47

195. Gilchrist, J. M., Moore, M. B., Andres, A., Estroff, J. A. & Badger, T. M. Ultrasonographic patterns of reproductive organs in infants fed soy formula: comparisons to infants fed breast milk and milk formula. *The Journal of pediatrics* **156,** 215–220; 10.1016/j.jpeds.2009.08.043 (2010).

196. Andres, A. *et al.* Compared with feeding infants breast milk or cow-milk formula, soy formula feeding does not affect subsequent reproductive organ size at 5 years of age. *The Journal of nutrition* **145,** 871–875; 10.3945/jn.114.206201 (2015).

197. Adgent, M. A. *et al.* A Longitudinal Study of Estrogen-Responsive Tissues and Hormone Concentrations in Infants Fed Soy Formula. *The Journal of clinical endocrinology and metabolism* **103,** 1899–1909; 10.1210/jc.2017-02249 (2018).

198. Upson, K., Adgent, M. A., Wegienka, G. & Baird, D. D. Soy-based infant formula feeding and menstrual pain in a cohort of women aged 23-35 years. *Human reproduction (Oxford, England)* **34,** 148–154; 10.1093/humrep/dey303 (2019).

199. Mori, F. *et al.* A kwashiorkor case due to the use of an exclusive rice milk diet to treat atopic dermatitis. *Nutrition journal* **14,** 83; 10.1186/s12937-015-0071-7 (2015).

200. Weaver, G. *et al.* Recommendations for the Establishment and Operation of Human Milk Banks in Europe: A Consensus Statement From the European Milk Bank Association (EMBA). *Frontiers in pediatrics* **7,** 53; 10.3389/fped.2019.00053 (2019).

201. AAP. Donor Human Milk for the High-Risk Infant: Preparation, Safety, and Usage Options in the United States. *Pediatrics* **139**; 10.1542/peds.2016-3440 (2017).

202. Scott, J., Ahwong, E., Devenish, G., Ha, D. & Do, L. Determinants of Continued Breastfeeding at 12 and 24 Months: Results of an Australian Cohort Study. *IJERPH* **16**; 10.3390/ijerph16203980 (2019).

203. WHO. Infant and young child feeding. Available at https://www.who.int/news-room/fact-sheets/detail/infant-and-young-child-feeding (2018).

204. Chowdhury, R. *et al.* Breastfeeding and maternal health outcomes: a systematic review and meta-analysis. *Acta paediatrica (Oslo, Norway : 1992)* **104,** 96–113; 10.1111/apa.13102 (2015).

205. Kramer, M. S. & Kakuma, R. Optimal duration of exclusive breastfeeding. *The Cochrane database of systematic reviews,* CD003517; 10.1002/14651858.CD003517.pub2 (2012).

206. Grizzo, F. M. F. *et al.* How does women's bone health recover after lactation? A systematic review and meta-analysis. *Osteoporosis international : a journal established as result of cooperation between the European Foundation for Osteoporosis and the National Osteoporosis Foundation of the USA* **31,** 413–427; 10.1007/s00198-019-05236-8 (2020).

207. Abou-Dakn, M. Gesundheitliche Auswirkungen des Stillens auf die Mutter. *Bundesgesundheitsblatt, Gesundheitsforschung, Gesundheitsschutz* **61,** 986–989; 10.1007/s00103-018-2776-1 (2018).
208. Verduci, E. *et al.* Cow's Milk Substitutes for Children: Nutritional Aspects of Milk from Different Mammalian Species, Special Formula and Plant-Based Beverages. *Nutrients* **11**; 10.3390/nu11081739 (2019).
209. Hojsak, I. *et al.* Arsenic in rice: a cause for concern. *Journal of pediatric gastroenterology and nutrition* **60,** 142–145; 10.1097/MPG.0000000000000502 (2015).
210. Keller, M. D., Shuker, M., Heimall, J. & Cianferoni, A. Severe malnutrition resulting from use of rice milk in food elimination diets for atopic dermatitis. *The Israel Medical Association journal : IMAJ* **14,** 40–42 (2012).
211. Daniels, L. A. Feeding Practices and Parenting: A Pathway to Child Health and Family Happiness. *Annals of nutrition & metabolism* **74 Suppl 2,** 29–42; 10.1159/000499145 (2019).
212. Jansen, P. W. *et al.* Using Food to Soothe in Infancy is Prospectively Associated with Childhood BMI in a Population-Based Cohort. *The Journal of nutrition* **149,** 788–794; 10.1093/jn/nxy277 (2019).
213. Abraham, K., Buhrke, T. & Lampen, A. Bioavailability of cyanide after consumption of a single meal of foods containing high levels of cyanogenic glycosides: a crossover study in humans. *Archives of toxicology* **90,** 559–574; 10.1007/s00204-015-1479-8 (2016).

This page is dedicated to you.

Index

51

Printed in Great Britain
by Amazon

75090527R00040